miracle juices™

immune

boosters

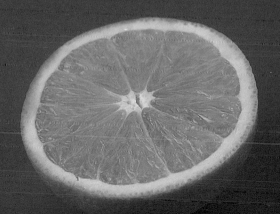

Safety Note

Immune Boosters should not be considered a replacement for
professional medical treatment; a physician should be consulted
on all matters relating to health. While the advice and information
in this book is believed to be accurate, the publisher cannot
accept any legal responsibility or liability for any injury or illness
sustained while following the advice in this book.

First published in Great Britain in 2002 by Hamlyn,
a division of Octopus Publishing Group Ltd
2–4 Heron Quays, London E14 4JP

Copyright © Octopus Publishing Group Ltd 2002

ISBN 0 600 60673 2

A CIP catalogue record for this book is available
from the British Library

Printed and bound in China

10 9 8 7 6 5 4 3 2 1

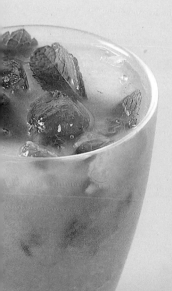

Contents

introduction

Is your immune system suffering?

Do you catch every bug that is being passed around the office or at home? Are you always sniffling and sneezing? If the answer is yes, your biggest ally in the fight against sickness is a strong immune system. Building up your immunity will not only help you resist disease now, but also lower your chances of suffering from chronic illnesses in later life.

We are surrounded by germs every day of our lives and the human body can be very resourceful in dealing with them. It has a whole host of tricks to fight off viruses, bacteria and other unwanted visitors. But if you aren't eating a balanced diet containing the correct proportions of certain vitamins and minerals, then the immune system will take a tumble, and all those germs will be able to get a hold on the body.

How the immune system works

- The skin, stomach acid, friendly bacteria in the gut, urine and tears act as a first line of defence against unwanted germs.
- White blood cells called lymphocytes travel around the body on the look out for any bacteria, viruses or other infecting agents. Once they have found a foreign body, they produce antibodies and toxins that will exterminate it.
- Monocytes and macrophages (other forms of white blood cells) encompass any germs that are found and digest them. You will know this is happening when inflammation occurs.

How to boost the immune system

There are ten key nutrients which

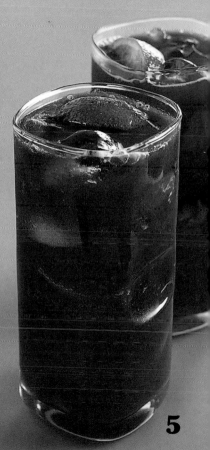

immune system: vitamin A, beta-carotene, vitamin B complex, vitamin C, vitamin E, calcium, selenium, zinc, iron and magnesium. Collectively, they support the immune system by:

- Acting as powerful antioxidants, antiviral and antibacterial agents, and antihistamines. Antioxidants protect the body against damage by free radicals, which can cause degenerative disease.
- Maintaining the lymphatic system and helping in the production of white blood cells and antibodies.
- Helping convert essential fatty acids into anti-inflammatory prostaglandins. Without prostaglandins, the body couldn't regulate the activity of the white blood cells, which would lead to more colds, infections and allergies.
- Guarding against the damage caused by pollution.

5

phytonutrients

Recent research has unearthed a whole new set of compounds that, although not classed as essential to life, can have a very positive impact on our health. These are known as phytonutrients and there are well over a hundred different types.

They are powerful antioxidants that work hand in hand with vitamins and minerals to keep degenerative diseases at bay and maintain a healthy immune system.

The simplest way to ensure you are preparing food rich in these compounds is to include naturally colourful fruits, vegetables and even seaweed in your diet.

Where to find phytonutrients

- Lycopene is found in red food, primarily tomatoes.
- Curcumin is present in yellow food, such as corn and yellow peppers.
- Anthoxanthins are also found in yellow foods. Potatoes and yellow-skinned onions are good sources.
- Carotenoids are of particular benefit to the immune system. Any foods in the orange spectrum will provide them. Eat plenty of cantaloupe melon, papaya, mangoes, carrots, apricots and squash.
- Anthocyanidins and proanthocyanidins come cloaked in the colours purple or blue. Raise your intake of blueberries, blackberries, black cherries, black grapes, blackcurrants, beetroot and cranberries.

- Chlorophyll promotes quick healing and guards against diseases such as cancer. Wherever you see green, you'll find it. Include some of these every day: cabbage, broccoli, kale, salad leaves, seaweed, wheatgrass and algae such spirulina.

top tips

- The B vitamins and vitamin C readily dissolve in water, so when cooking vegetables or brown rice, use the cooking water in the finished meal as it is a concentrated source of vitamins.
- Drink fresh juices soon after making them as many vitamins degrade quickly on contact with air.
- Vitamins A and C are easily perishable in the human body, so your intake should be spread throughout the day for maximum benefit.
- Key sources of antioxidants are all orange, red, purple, yellow and green fruits and vegetables, potatoes, nuts, seeds, wheatgerm, garlic and onions, shellfish, poultry, whole grains, liver, eggs, lean meat and full-fat dairy produce.
- Key sources of essential fatty acids include cold-pressed oils, nuts, seeds and oily fish.
- In a world where food processing is sapping the goodness out of wholesome natural foods and our eating habits leave a lot to be desired, vitamin and mineral supplements may be required. Always consult a qualified nutritionist to identify what you may be lacking before embarking on a supplement program.

top ten nutrients

Nutrient	Actions	Best Source	Recommended daily dosage
Vitamin A	Antioxidant; metabolizes fatty acids; fight colds and infections; maintains mucous membranes; maintains the thymus gland.	Liver, eggs, full-fat dairy produce, cod liver oil, oily fish.	4000–10,000 iu
Beta-carotene	Converted into vitamin A in the body.	Butternut squash, pumpkin, melon, sweet potatoes, carrots, apricots, mangoes, green leafy vegetables.	4000–10000 iu
Vitamin B complex	Vitamins B6 and B3 help convert essential fatty acids into anti-inflammatory prostaglandins. B5 is required for antibody production and maintains the white blood cells.	Whole grains, liver, poultry, game, wheatgerm, brewers yeast.	B1: 1.5 mg, B2: 1.7 mg, B3: 20 mg, B6: 2 mg, B12: 6 mcg
Vitamin C	Helps absorb calcium, iron and certain amino acids; enables the body to excrete poisonous substances; increases immune response; has antihistamine properties; helps prevent anaemia; speeds up the healing process of wounds; a powerful antioxidant.	Broccoli, parsley, kiwi fruit, citrus fruit, berries, peppers, blackcurrants, Brussels sprouts, papaya, mangoes.	100 mg minimum. Many nutritionists recommend 1500–4000 mg
Vitamin E	Powerful antioxidant; helps pituitary hormone production; assists cellular regeneration; guards against pollutants; accelerates healing; inhibits carcinogens; helps antibody response to infection.	Avocado, nuts, seeds, unrefined oils, wheatgerm, oatmeal.	12–15 iu minimum. 100–600 iu is recommended by nutritionists.

Nutrient	Actions	Best Source	Recommended daily dosage
Calcium	Vital for the bones and phagocytic cells; helps the metabolism of essential fatty acids.	Dairy products, fortified soya products, nuts, seeds, tinned fish with bones, dark green vegetables.	800–1200 mg
Magnesium	Activates metabolic enzymes; helps utilize vitamins C and E, helps convert glucose to energy; necessary for antibody production.	Nuts, seeds, green leafy vegetables, root vegetables, egg yolks, whole grains, dried fruit.	350–450 mg
Iron	Vital for formation of haemoglobin and white blood cells and antibodies; relieves fatigue; prevents anaemia; promotes immune system; and aids growth.	Liver, red meat, eggs, whole grains, green leafy vegetables, beans, lentils, nuts, seeds, blackstrap molasses.	10–18 mg
Zinc	Essential for the immune system; vital for the production of white blood cells, especially the lymphocytes; metabolizes essential fatty acids; lowers histamine production; accelerates healing; helps form insulin; increases overall natural immunity.	Shellfish, poultry, game, lean red meat, pulses, seeds, nuts, whole grains.	15–40 mg
Selenium	A powerful antioxidant; helps in the production of antibodies.	Nuts, seeds, whole grains, seafood.	50–200 mcg

why juice?

Vital vitamins and minerals such as antioxidants, vitamins A, B, C and E, folic acid, potassium, calcium, magnesium, zinc and amino acids are present in fresh fruits and vegetables, and are all necessary for optimum health. Because juicing removes the indigestible fibre in fruits and vegetables, the nutrients are available to the body in much larger quantities than if the piece of fruit or vegetable were eaten whole. For example, when you eat a raw carrot you are able to assimilate only about 1 per cent of the available beta-carotene, because many of the nutrients are trapped in the fibre. When a carrot is juiced, thereby removing the fibre, nearly 100 per cent of the beta-carotene can be assimilated. Juicing several types of fruits and vegetables on a daily basis is therefore an easy way to ensure that your body receives its

full quota of vitamins and minerals.

In addition, fruits and vegetables provide another substance absolutely essential for good health — water. Most people don't consume enough water. In fact, many of the fluids we drink — coffee, tea, soft drinks, alcoholic beverages and artificially flavoured drinks — contain substances that require extra water for the body to eliminate, and tend to be dehydrating. Fruit and vegetable juices are free of these unnecessary substances.

Your health

A diet high in fruits and vegetables can prevent and help to cure a wide range of ailments. At the cutting edge of nutritional research are the plant chemicals known as phytochemicals, which hold the key to preventing deadly diseases such as cancer and heart disease, and others such as asthma, arthritis and allergies.

Although juicing benefits your overall health, it should be used only to complement your daily eating plan. You must still eat enough from the other food groups (such as grains, dairy food and pulses) to ensure your body maintains strong bones and healthy cells. If you are following a specially prescribed diet, or are under medical supervision, do discuss any drastic changes with your health practitioner before beginning any type of new health regime.

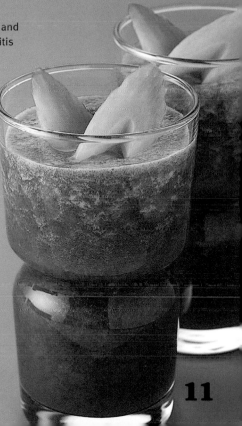

how to juice

Available in a variety of models, juicers work by separating the fruit and vegetable juice from the pulp. Choose a juicer with a reputable brand name, that has an opening big enough for larger fruits and vegetables, and make sure it is easy to take apart and clean, otherwise you may become discouraged from using it.

Types of juicer

A citrus juicer, or lemon squeezer is ideal for extracting the juice from oranges, lemons, limes and grapefruit, especially if you want to add just a small amount of citrus juice to another liquid. Pure citrus juice has a high acid content, which may upset or irritate your stomach, so is best diluted with water.

Centrifugal juicers are the most widely used and affordable juicers on the market. Fresh fruits and vegetables are fed into a rapidly spinning grater, and the pulp separated from the juice by centrifugal force. The pulp is retained in the machine while the juice runs into a separate jug. A centrifugal juicer produces less juice than the more expensive masticating juicer, which works by pulverizing fruits and

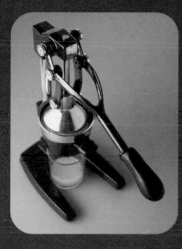

of one part white vinegar to two parts water will lessen any staining from the fruits and vegetables.

Preparing produce for juicing

Prepare ingredients just before juicing so that fewer nutrients are lost through oxidization. Cut or tear foods into manageable pieces for juicing. If the ingredients are not organic, do not include stems, skins or roots, but if the produce is organic, you can put everything in the juicer. However, don't include the skins from pineapple, mango, papaya, citrus fruit and banana; and remove the stones from avocados, apricots, peaches, mangoes and plums. You can include melon seeds, particularly watermelon, as these are full of juice. For grape juice, choose green grapes with an amber tinge or black grapes with a darkish bloom. Leave the pith on lemons for the pectin content.

vegetables and pushing them through a wire mesh with immense force.

Cleaning the juicer

Clean your juicing machine thoroughly – a toothbrush or nailbrush works well for removing stubborn residual pulp. Soaking the equipment in warm soapy water will loosen the residue from those hard-to-reach places. A solution

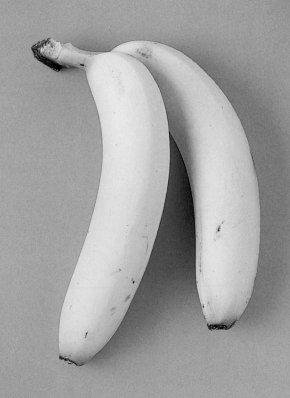

heal

This drink is bursting with beta-carotene, which is converted into vitamin A in the body.

lift-off

100 g (3½ oz) red pepper
125 g (4 oz) strawberries
50 g (2 oz) tomato
125 g (4 oz) mango
125 g (4 oz) watermelon
3 ice cubes
mango slices, to decorate
  (optional)

Juice all the ingredients, whizz in a blender or food processor with the ice cubes and serve in a tall glass. Decorate with mango slices, if liked.

Makes 200 ml (7 fl oz)

Nutritional Values

- Kcals: 200
- vitamin A: 9630 iu
- vitamin C: 231 mg
- selenium: 2.66 mcg
- zinc: 0.58 mg

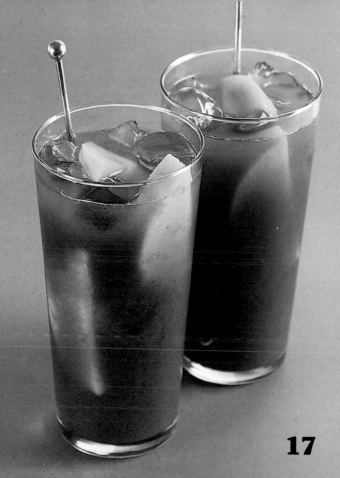

17

Spinach is a useful source of iron. It also contains good amounts of vitamins C, E, B1 and B6, and folic acid.

iron maiden

large handful of baby spinach
200 g (7 oz) carrot
4 tomatoes
½ red pepper
ice cubes

Juice the vegetables in alternating batches to ensure the spinach leaves do not clog the juicer. Pour the juice into a glass and add a couple of ice cubes.
Makes 300 ml (½ pint)

Nutritional Values

- Kcals: 175
- vitamin A: 71065 iu
- vitamin C: 208 mg
- vitamin E: 3.33 mg
- iron: 3.8 mg
- calcium: 169 mg

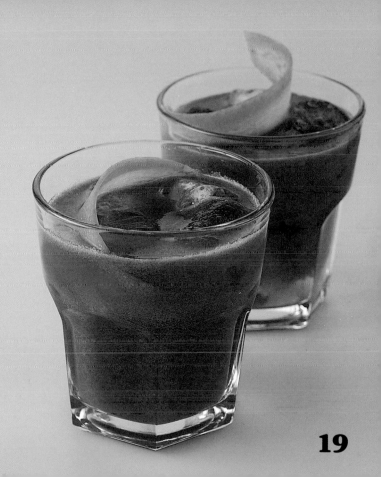

19

Carrots, beetroot and oranges are all high in vitamins A and C, antioxidants and phytonutrients. This juice is also a rich source of potassium. A real tonic.

power pack

1 orange
250 g (8 oz) carrot
125 g (4 oz) beetroot
ice cubes
125 g (4 oz) strawberries
orange rind, to decorate
** (optional)**

Peel the orange, leaving on as much pith as possible. Juice the carrot, beetroot and orange. Put the juice into a blender or food processor with a couple of ice cubes and the strawberries. Whizz for 20 seconds and serve in a tall glass. Decorate with strips of orange rind, if liked.
Makes 200 ml (7 fl oz)

Nutritional Values

- Kcals: 259
- vitamin A: 70652 iu
- vitamin C: 166 mg
- potassium: 1646 mg
- magnesium: 91.5 mg
- selenium: 5.1 mcg

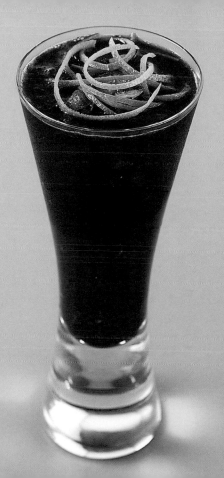

21

A juice rich in antioxidants. The lime encourages the elimination of toxins.

ginger zinger

125 g (4 oz) carrot
250 g (8 oz) cantaloupe
  melon
1 lime
2.5 cm (1 inch) cube
  fresh root ginger,
  roughly chopped
ice cubes

To decorate:
lime wedges
cardamom seeds

Juice the carrot, melon, lime and ginger.
Serve in a glass over ice. Decorate
with lime wedges and seeds from a
cardamom pod.
Makes 200 ml (7 fl oz)

Nutritional Values

- Kcals: 166
- vitamin A: 4262 iu
- vitamin C: 137 mg
- selenium: 2.7 mcg
- zinc: 0.84 mg

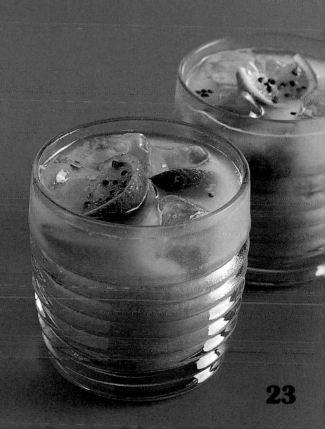

23

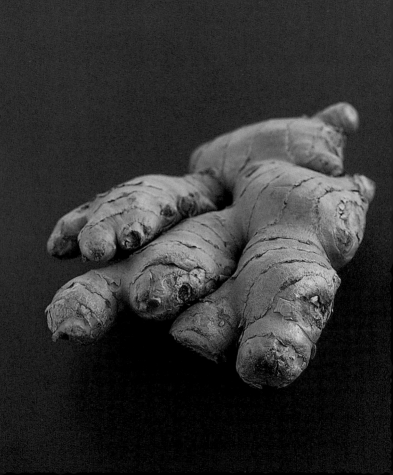

fortify

Papaya helps to calm the digestive system; cucumber flushes out toxins and orange gives a great boost of vitamin C. The overall effect is calming and rehydrating.

morning after

**125 g (4 oz) papaya
2 oranges
125 g (4 oz) cucumber
ice cubes**

**To decorate:
cucumber slices
papaya slices**

Peel the papaya and the oranges, leaving on as much pith as possible. Juice them together with the cucumber and serve in a tall glass over ice. Decorate with slices of cucumber and papaya.
Makes 200 ml (7 fl oz)

Nutritional Values

- Kcals: 184
- vitamin A: 1123 iu
- vitamin C: 218 mg
- magnesium: 51 mg
- potassium: 1004 mg
- selenium: 2 mcg

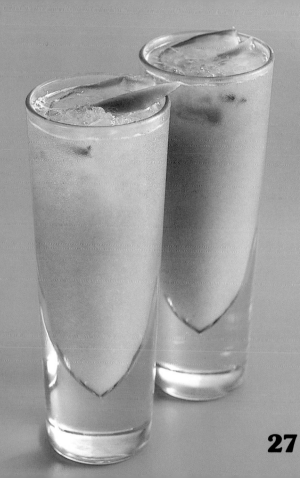

27

All the ingredients in this juice have antibacterial properties.
It is particularly effective if you are taking antibiotics.

live and kicking

250 g (8 oz) apple
100 g (3½ oz) frozen cranberries
100 g (3½ oz) live natural yogurt
1 tablespoon clear honey
ice cubes

Juice the apple and whizz in a blender or food processor with the cranberries, yogurt and honey. Serve in a tumbler over ice cubes.
Makes 200 ml (7 fl oz)

Nutritional Values

- Kcals: 339
- vitamin C: 20 mg
- calcium: 40 mg
- magnesium: 25 mg
- zinc: 1.7 mg

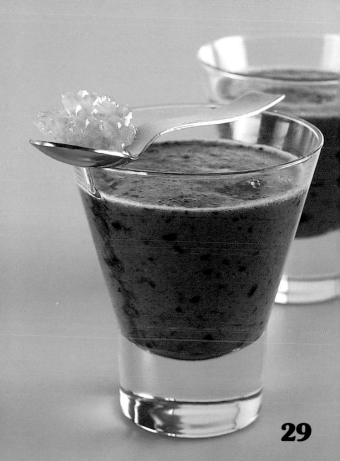

29

This juice is another good choice if you're run down and fighting the winter round of colds and flu. Peppers are a favourite for warding off infection, and are also natural painkillers.

sergeant pep-up

1 orange
100 g (3½ oz) red pepper
100 g (3½ oz) yellow pepper
100 g (3½ oz) orange pepper
ice cubes
1 tablespoon mint leaves, plus extra to decorate

Peel the orange, leaving on as much pith as possible. Juice the peppers and orange and serve in a tumbler with ice cubes. Stir in the mint and decorate with mint leaves, if liked.
Makes 200 ml (7 fl oz)

Nutritional Values

- Kcals: 141
- vitamin A: 2146 iu
- vitamin C: 333 mg
- selenium: 1.52 mcg
- zinc: 0.44 mg

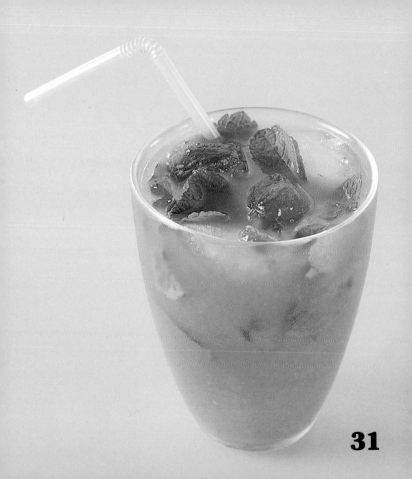

31

A sharp clean-tasting drink full of vitamin A and vitamin C, selenium and zinc.

'c' red

150 g (5 oz) grapefruit
50 g (2 oz) kiwi fruit
175 g (6 oz) pineapple
50 g (2 oz) frozen
  raspberries
50 g (2 oz) frozen
  cranberries

Juice the grapefruit, kiwi and pineapple.
Whizz in a blender with the frozen berries.
Decorate with a few extra raspberries and
serve with straws.
Makes 200 ml (7 fl oz)

Nutritional Values

- Kcals: 247
- vitamin A: 693 iu
- vitamin C: 179 mg
- selenium: 4.3 mcg
- zinc: 1.43 mg

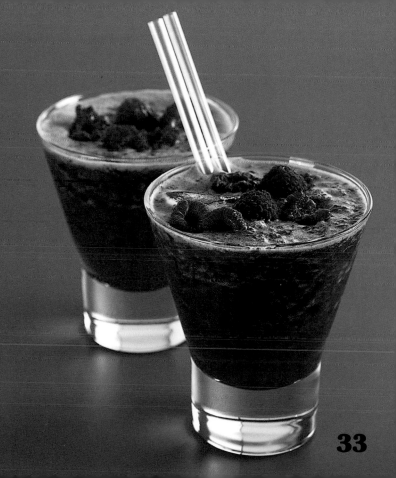

33

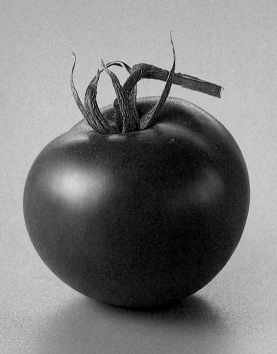

protect

This juice is rich in vitamin C, which is great for fighting off bronchial illness. Enzymes in the pineapple dissolve mucus, and the chilli is a great expectorant. Chillies are rich in carotenoids and vitamin C, and are thought to help increase blood flow. They also have antibacterial properties, which make them a favourite for beating colds and flu.

chill buster

250 g (8 oz) carrot
½ small deseeded chilli or a sprinkling of chilli powder
250 g (8 oz) pineapple
ice cubes
½ lime
1 tablespoon chopped coriander leaves

Juice the carrot, chilli and pineapple. Serve in a tall glass over ice cubes. Squeeze in the lime juice and stir in the chopped coriander leaves to serve.
Makes 200 ml (7 fl oz)

Nutritional Values

- Kcals: 240
- vitamin A: 70382 iu
- vitamin C: 72 mg
- selenium: 3.95 mcg
- zinc: 0.73 mg

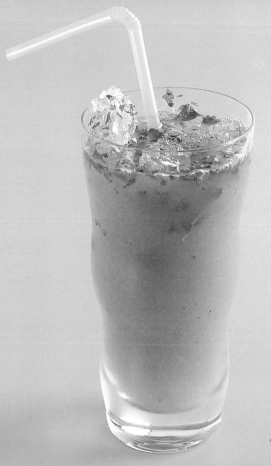

37

If you're run down and haven't been eating a balanced diet, your immune system becomes more susceptible to colds and flu. At the first sign of symptoms, drinking juices with papaya, lemon, lime, garlic or ginger may help.

frisky sour

150 g (5 oz) papaya
150 g (5 oz) grapefruit
150 g (5 oz) raspberries
½ lime
ice cubes
lime slices, to decorate

Scoop out the flesh of the papaya, and juice it with the grapefruit (with the pith left on), and the raspberries. Squeeze in the lime juice and mix. Serve with a few ice cubes and decorate with lime slices.
Makes 200 ml (7 fl oz)

Nutritional Values

- Kcals: 193
- vitamin A: 810 iu
- vitamin C: 188 mg
- selenium: 4.05 mcg
- zinc: 1.09 mg

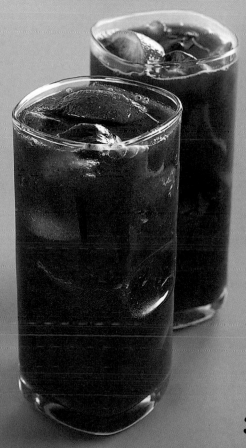

39

Tomatoes and carrots provide large amounts of vitamin C, ideal for maintaining a healthy body. Garlic, ginger and horseradish are all powerful antioxidants – imperative for fighting off infections. Combined, they also deal a mighty anti-mucus punch.

hot stuff

300 g (10 oz) tomato
100 g (3½ oz) celery
2.5 cm (1 inch) cube
fresh root ginger,
roughly chopped
1 garlic clove
2.5 cm (1 inch) cube
fresh horseradish
175 g (6 oz) carrot
2 ice cubes
celery slivers, to decorate
(optional)

Juice all the ingredients, whizz the juice in a blender or food processor with the ice cubes and serve in a tumbler. Decorate with celery slivers, if liked.
Makes 150 ml (¼ pint)

Nutritional Values

• Kcals: 189
• vitamin A: 51253 iu
• vitamin C: 87 mg
• selenium: 4.47 mcg
• zinc: 5.52 mg

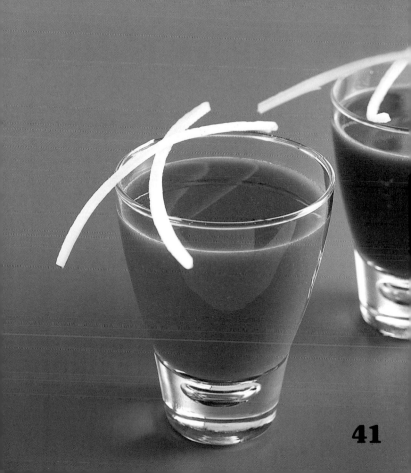

41

This simple and quenching juice is bursting with vitamin C and betacarotene, making it an invaluable immune booster.

red-hot remedy

4 large tomatoes
1 apple
1 celery stick
ice cubes
4 basil leaves, finely chopped
1½ tablespoons lime juice

Juice the tomatoes, apple and celery. Pour into a glass over ice, and stir in the basil and lime juice.
Makes 200 ml (7 fl oz)

Nutritional Values

• Kcals: 203
• vitamin A: 5718 iu
• magnesium: 63 mg
• zinc: 0.6 mg

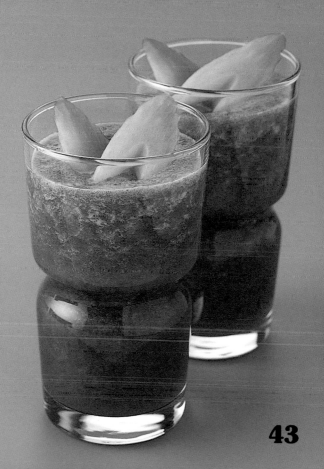

43

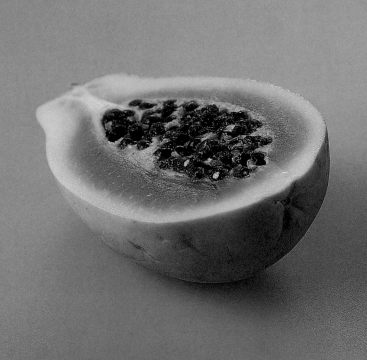

defend

This juice is full of vitamin C and phytonutrients, such as anthocyanidins, to help resist disease.

tummy tickler

300 g (10 oz) apple
200 g (7 oz)
   blackcurrants
ice cubes

Juice the fruit and serve over ice for a great blackcurrant cordial substitute. Decorate with extra blackcurrants, if liked.
Makes 200 ml (7 fl oz)

Nutritional Values

- Kcals: 300
- vitamin C: 415 mg
- calcium: 30 mg

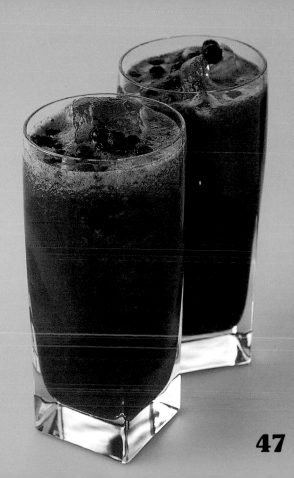

47

This juice cleanses the whole system: blood, kidneys and lymph.
The pectin in the apples strengthens the immune system.

bumpy
ride

200 g (7 oz) apple
50 g (2 oz) beetroot
90 g (3 oz) celery
ice cubes
apple slices, to decorate
   (optional)

Juice together the apple, beetroot and celery and serve over ice in a tumbler. Decorate with apple slices, if liked.
Makes 150 ml (¼ pint)

Nutritional Values

- Kcals: 179
- vitamin A: 480 iu
- vitamin C: 23 mg
- potassium: 763 mg
- magnesium: 37 mg

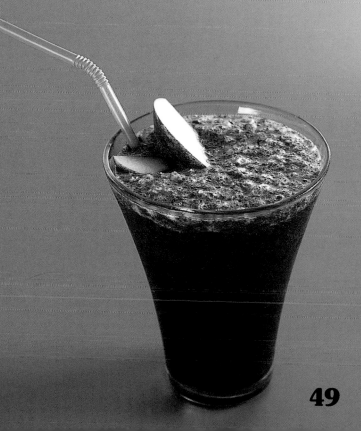

49

This juice packs a mighty antiviral punch, as it is bursting with vitamin C.

calm seas

2 oranges
1 kiwi fruit
200 g (7 oz) strawberries

Peel the oranges, leaving on as much pith as possible. Juice the oranges, kiwi fruit and strawberries, reserving some strawberries for decoration. Serve immediately.
Makes 200 ml (7 fl oz)

Nutritional Values

• Kcals: 201
• vitamin A: 726 iu
• vitamin C: 403 mg
• magnesium: 70 mg
• zinc: 0.8 mg

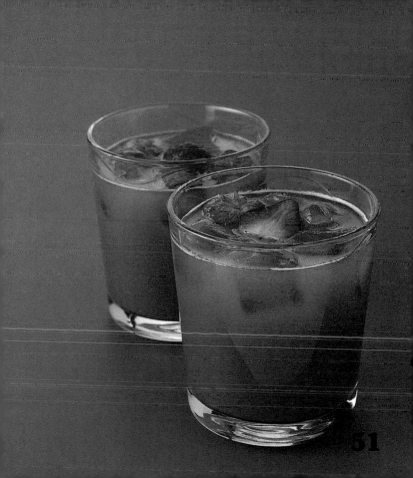

51

Full of iron, calcium and potassium, this is an all-round booster that is great for bones and teeth and keeping colds at bay.

top banana

100 g (3½ oz) orange
150 g (5 oz) carrot
100 g (3½ oz) banana
1 dried apricot
ice cubes
banana chunks, to decorate (optional)

Peel the orange, leaving on as much pith as possible. Juice the carrot and orange. Whizz in a blender or food processor with the banana, apricot and some ice cubes. Decorate with chunks of banana, if liked.
Makes 200 ml (7 fl oz)

Nutritional Values

- Kcals: 204
- vitamin A: 44570 iu
- vitamin C: 88 mg
- calcium: 101 mg
- potassium: 1475 mg
- iron: 2.5 mg

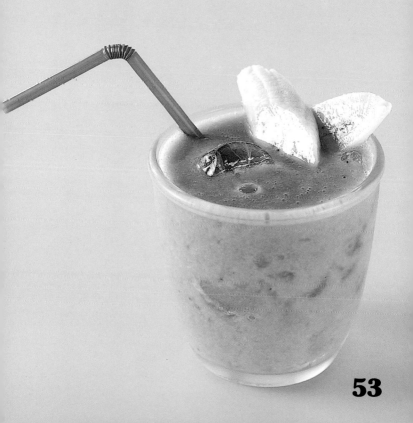

53

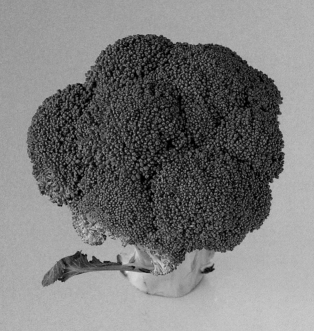

strengthen

This juice is an excellent source of vitamins A, C, B1, B6 and potassium.
In addition to being a natural remedy for travel sickness and morning sickness,
ginger is also believed to aid digestion and help the body fight off colds.

pick-me-up

200 g (7 oz) carrot
1 tart-flavoured apple,
  such as Granny Smith
1 cm (½ inch) cube fresh
  root ginger
ice cubes

Juice the carrots with the apple
and ginger. Pour into a glass and
add a couple of ice cubes.
Makes 250 ml (8 fl oz)

Nutritional Values

- Kcals: 127
- vitamin A: 60833 iu
- vitamin C: 30 mg
- iron: 0.9 mg
- calcium: 59 mg

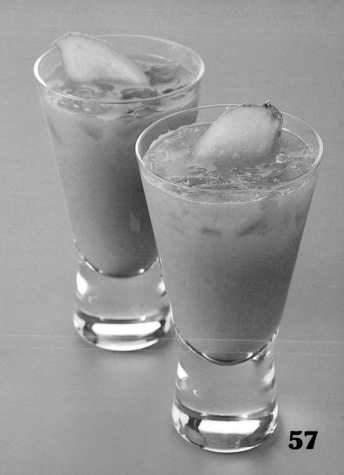

High in selenium, this is an ideal juice for smokers as it helps guard against lung cancer.

what's up broc?

250 g (8 oz) broccoli
175 g (6 oz) carrot
50 g (2 oz) beetroot
coriander sprig, to
    decorate (optional)

Juice all the ingredients and serve in a tall glass. Decorate with a coriander sprig, if liked.
Makes 200 ml (7 fl oz)

Nutritional Values

- Kcals: 172
- vitamin A: 52304 iu
- vitamin C: 43 mg
- selenium: 9.86 mcg
- zinc: 1.6 mg

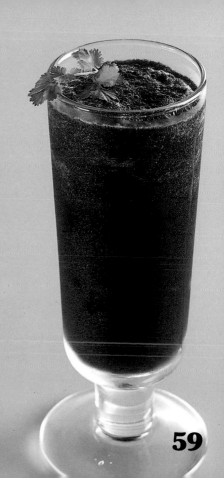

59

This juice is full of vitamins A and C, which should help keep colds at bay. Citrus fruits are also great mucus reducers.

vitamin vitality

2 oranges
125 g (4 oz) carrot

Peel the oranges, leaving on as much pith as possible. Juice the carrots with the oranges. Serve immediately.
Makes 200 ml (7 fl oz)

Nutritional Values

- Kcals: 188
- vitamin A: 34293 iu
- vitamin C: 151 mg
- magnesium: 44 mg
- zinc: 0.4 mg

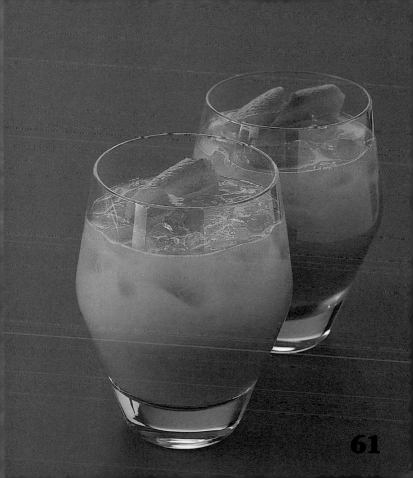

61

This juice has a high vitamin C content to ward off colds.
Strawberries are natural painkillers.

strawberry soother

200 g (7 oz) orange
200 g (7 oz) strawberries
ice cubes

Peel the orange, leaving on as much pith as possible. Juice the strawberries and orange, reserving some strawberries for decoration. Serve straight over ice, or whizz in a blender or food processor with a couple of ice cubes for a thicker drink.
Makes 200 ml (7 fl oz)

Nutritional Values

• Kcals: 154
• vitamin C: 219 mg
• potassium: 694 mg
• calcium: 108 mg

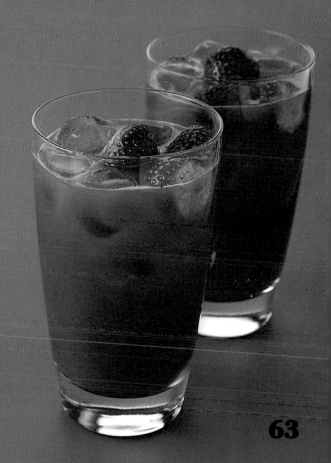

63

index

acknowledgements

The publisher would like to thank The Juicer Company for the loan of the Champion juicer and the Orange X citrus juicer (featured on pages 12 and 13).

The Juicer Company
28 Shambles
York
YO1 7LX
Tel: (01904) 541541
www.thejuicercompany.co.uk

Executive Editor Nicola Hill
Editor Camilla James
Executive Art Editor Geoff Fennell
Designer Sue Michniewicz
Senior Production Controller Jo Sim
Photographer Stephen Conroy
Home Economist David Morgan
Stylist Angela Swaffield
All photographs © Octopus Publishing Group Ltd